ISBN: 9781086667257

301 Healthy Living Tips

Weight Loss, Weight Maintenance, Healthy Eating & Fitness Tips

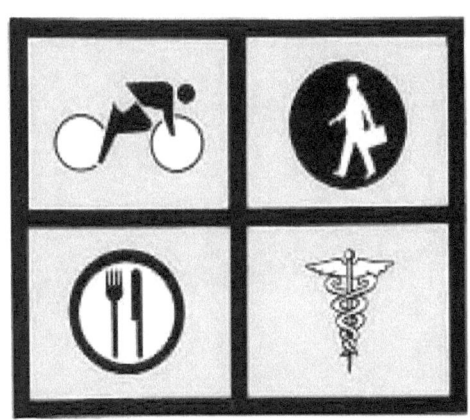

Compiled by NoPaperPress staff

Table of Contents

Weight Loss Tips

Probably the best thing you can do for your overall health is to lose weight. The following tips are offered to help you do just that in a healthy and natural way. Use the tips that apply to you and can best help you succeed. Good luck!

1) A reducing diet is best supervised by a physician. This is especially true when a great deal of weight needs to be lost, or if you have an ailment or a history of medical problems.

2) Understand that the only sure way to slim down for keeps is to eat less and exercise more. There are no safe short cuts or miracle methods for taking off weight.

3) Successful weight loss and subsequent weight maintenance requires knowledge, desire and discipline. Avoid the latest fad diets. Instead, take the time to develop a true understanding of weight control and then change your eating and activity habits accordingly.

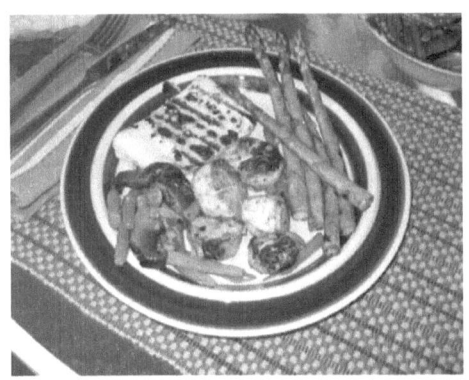

4) Consistently choose healthy foods, avoid harmful foods and large portions and exercise regularly. Nothing else will work over the long haul.

5) What constitutes a good reducing diet? A

good weight loss diet must provide you with an understanding of weight control as well as the knowledge you need to reduce your weight to the desired level.

6) A good reducing diet must also help you remain healthy while you are losing weight.

7) In addition, a good reducing diet must lead you to a healthier way of eating and exercising that will help you, in the long term, keep off the weight you have lost.

8) First, ask yourself: "Why am I overweight?" What are the main reasons? Do you eat too much of everything? Too much dessert? Drink too much beer? Is your only exercise walking from the TV to the fridge? Determine the why and then focus on those one or two problem areas. Sometimes it's that simple.

9) Experts agree that whether you are trying to lose weight or just maintain your weight, it's calories that count.   It doesn't matter what foods the calories are from – to lose weight you must eat fewer calories than you burn. Calories count!   Not carbs, not Weight Watchers points. Calories – period!

10) Weight control can be thought of as supply and demand. You lose weight if you supply your body with fewer calories than your activities demand. (In this case, your body uses energy you stored as fat to make up the calorie difference.)

11) Weight loss occurs when your food energy intake is less than the total energy you expend. This difference in calories is referred to as your calorie deficit.

12) How much weight you lose depends on the magnitude of your calorie deficit. To lose one pound requires a deficit of approximately 3,500 Calories.

13) Use Body Mass Index, or BMI, to determine what you should weigh. Your BMI is calculated by dividing your weight in kilograms by the square of your height in meters. (See "Weight Control – U.S. Edition," published by NoPaperPress.com for a convenient, easy-to-use chart).

14) Given two people the same age, gender and activity level, and on the same reducing diet, the heavier person will lose weight faster than the thinner person.

15) Given a male and female, the same age, weight, activity level and on the same reducing diet, the man will lose weight faster than the woman. This is due to the fact that women have less muscle and therefore lower basal metabolic rates than men. Hence, a woman must eat less than a man to lose the same amount of weight.

16) Given two individuals, the same gender, weight and activity level, the younger person will lose weight faster than the older person.

17) If your caloric intake is constant over the years you will slowly gain weight as you age. This is because your basal metabolic rate decreases as you advance in age, and most people tend not to be as active as they get older.

18) If you are overweight start on a weight loss diet now because it will only become more difficult to lose weight as you get older.

19) If your caloric intake on a weight-loss diet is constant, your rate of weight loss will decrease with time. So if you want to lose weight at a constant rate over time, you must eat slightly less (or exercise harder) as you lose weight.

20) Inevitably, everyone on a diet hits a exasperating weight-loss plateau. The only way to bust through the plateau is to reduce your caloric intake and/or to step up your exercise intensity.

21) Slow weight loss is healthier, is more likely to be permanent, and is easier to sustain over the long haul. So when it comes to weight loss, don't be in a hurry!

22) A very important weight-profile parameter is your waist-to-hip ratio. Health risks for heart attack and stroke increase considerably for men with a ratio above 1.0 and for women with a ratio above 0.8. To calculate your ratio, measure your waist size (at its narrowest circumference) and divide it by your hip size (at its widest section).

23) The general weight-loss rule is "last on first off." When you lose weight, it normally it will come off in the reverse order of where you gained it. And there is not much you can do about that. There is no food, no exercise, no magic pill that will cause your body to lose fat in one place rather than another.

24) To determine your frame size, circle your wrist with your thumb and third finger. If the tips of your fingers overlap, you have a small frame. If they just

touch you are medium, and if they don't touch you have a large frame.

26) An understanding of nutrition is not only vital for good health but will also help you control your weight in the long term.

27) Keep a daily food log to record everything you eat. For some people it really works wonders.

28) Read food labels carefully to know what's in the food you buy and eat, and to avoid foods with hidden calories.

29) "Eat Slowly." This is especially vital when you're trying to lose weight. If you're someone who eats fast, you're not giving yourself a chance to feel full. While everyone else is still eating, you either sit and pick, or you have seconds, taking in extra calories you could avoid if you would just slow down.

30) Drink lots of water – about 8 glasses per day. Try adding a slice of lemon to make it more interesting.   Often, when you think you're hungry, you're just thirsty. So, next time you reach for a snack, drink some water first and see if that does it for you.

31) Hunger is your body's way of telling you that you need fuel, that is calories. When you're done eating, you should feel satisfied – but not stuffed.

32) Remember your stomach is about the size of your fist. So it doesn't take much food to fill it comfortably.

33) All foods are a combination of water, carbohydrate, protein, fat and fiber. Knowing this

can lead to a better understanding of why a food has a particular caloric value.

34) When on a diet, an awareness of the caloric value (per ounce) of some basic foods can really be helpful.

35) Fat (lard) has the highest calorie per ounce value – about 260.   Sugar (a pure carbohydrate) at 110 Calories per ounce is near the middle of the calorie spectrum.

36) Water and fiber contain no calories – that is zero Calories per ounce.

37) One dilemma for dieters is judging portion size. It makes no sense to worry about whether a cut of lean meat has 70 or 80 Calories per ounce if you have no idea whether the portion you are eating weighs four or ten ounces. To be successful, learn to estimate portion sizes with reasonable accuracy.

38) Judging the weight of meat or poultry is one of the most important parts of any diet. As a guide, four ounces of meat or poultry is about the size of a slice of bread: 4 x 4 x ¼ inch.

39) To control portion size, that is the amount of food you eat, use a salad plate instead of a dinner plate.

40) Eat the low-cal items on your plate first. Start with a broth soup, then the salad and veggies. By the time you get to the higher calorie meat and starch you'll be almost full and will eat less of them.

41) Studies show people who eat 5 to 6 mini-meals and snacks a day don't feel as hungry and are better able to control their appetite and their weight.

42) Foods loaded with flavor stimulate your taste buds and are more satisfying. So add herbs and spices to
your food for a flavor boost and you might not eat as much.

43) When on a diet simple is better. Why? Because simple, uncomplicated meals usually contain fewer "hidden calories" than more elaborate dishes.

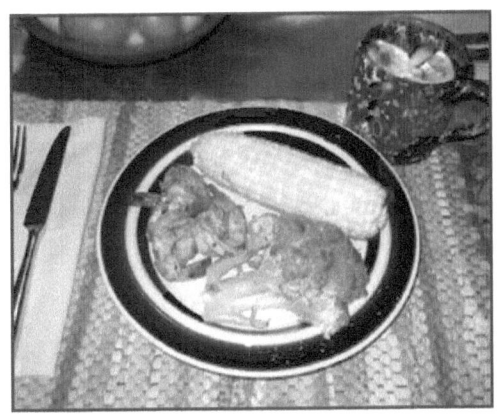

44) Fat-free isn't always your best bet.   Low fat doesn't necessarily mean low calorie! Most often sugar is substituted for fat and the calorie total remains the same or even higher. Instead, look for low-calorie or reduced-calorie foods.

45) Fat-free (skim) milk is the exception. To cut calories, switch to 1-percent milk or even better fat-free skim milk.

46) Hot or cold cereal topped with fruit, and fat-free milk makes a nutritious, relatively low-calorie meal anytime.

47) For a quick low-cal meal, try a peanut butter sandwich on whole wheat bread with a glass of 1-percent milk and an apple.

48) Keep several bags of your favorite frozen vegetables on hand. Mix any combination, microwave, and top with your favorite light salad dressing. Makes a great low-cal meal.

49) For another quick low-cal meal, try a Lean Cuisine, Smart Ones, or Healthy Choice frozen entree with a salad and a glass of un-sweet ice tea.

50) Keep lean sandwich fixings on hand (whole-wheat bread, sliced turkey, reduced-fat cheese, lettuce, tomatoes and mustard).

51) Try to use mustard on a sandwich instead of mayo.

52) For a healthy and relatively low-calorie meal, buy a veggie sandwich on whole-wheat bread at Subway.

53) If you hate veggies, eat plenty of fruit instead. Fruit is just about as healthy and low-calorie as vegetables.

54) To prevent a diet from becoming monotonous, after a few weeks try exchanging or substituting foods – a technique used by dieticians. Exchanging a food listed in a diet for another food with approximately equal caloric value and nutritional content is the foundation of a successful long-term diet.

55) Handle occasional overeating by compensating. To do this, estimate how far you have strayed from your weight-loss diet and then make amends at the next opportunity (usually the next meal or two) – by eating less.

56) Learn to change your eating habits to meet changing activity levels – that is don't eat as much when you're activity level declines.

57) Most nutritionists recommend that you eat a substantial breakfast because then you'll likely eat less the remainder of the day.

58) Eating late at night doesn't by itself cause weight gain. Because it's the total number of calories that count – not when you eat them.

59) But don't "snack" yourself fat. You can easily munch 600 calories of chips and dips while watching late-night TV.

60) A majority of people who struggle with night-binge eating are those who skip meals during the day. Make sure you eat breakfast, lunch, and dinner.

61) To avoid night-binge eating, change your evening routine. Rather than watching TV get into a hobby that will occupy your mind and hands.

62) Post a notice on your kitchen and refrigerator doors: "Closed After Dinner."

63) Brush your teeth immediately after dinner to discourage you from continued eating.

64) Eating in a restaurant can be a challenge because most restaurant portions are huge, and can easily total more than 1,500 Calories. So, when you're in a restaurant decide how much to eat – and take the remainder home. A good rule of thumb is to eat half and bring the rest home.

65) When you're eating out, consider ordering children's portions or a small sandwich as a way to trim calories and get the size of your meals under control.

66) In a restaurant, consider ordering two appetizers (one should be low-calorie) instead of an entrée, and always request sauces and dressings on the side.

67) For even better calorie control, eat at home rather than in a restaurant.

68) To save calories and money, instead of eating out, bring your lunch to work.

69) Before you go to a party, have a very small meal or snack to take the edge off your appetite and make it easier to resist high-calorie goodies.

70) At a party, don't stand near temptation – the food and the bar!   You'll probably eat and drink less.

71) If you host a dinner party, when company leaves, have them take some of the leftover food (particularly the dessert) with them – or take the leftovers to work the next day.

72) Beware of alcoholic beverages. Beer has about 13 Calories per ounce, wine has 25 Calories per ounce and whiskey has a whopping 71 Calories per ounce!

73) Drink alcoholic beverages in moderation and try to restrict any alcoholic drinking to weekends.

74) **Stop drinking your calories.** Alcoholic drinks, fancy coffees, regular soda, and even fruit juice are high in calories – but they don't make you feel full.

75) **Dilute fruit juices, such as apple juice, orange juice, etc. with water.** This does cut the flavor slightly but really reduces the calorie content.

76) **Don't have sweets in your home. This makes them easier to resist. Out of sight, out of mind!**

77) **Instead of sweets, for a delicious, healthy, low-calorie dessert have a low-cal smoothie, or sliced fruit over low-fat or fat-free yogurt.**

78) **On the other hand, not eating your favorite foods sometimes triggers "rebound" overeating. Even on a diet you can still enjoy your favorite foods – but do so in moderation.**

79) **If you must have sweets, allow about 150 calories per day for your favorite sweet which amounts to about one ounce of chocolate, half a** slice of cake, or ½ **cup of ice cream.**

81) **Steaming in a microwave is an excellent way to cook veggies so they retain nutrients. Another advantage is that steaming adds no fat (calories) or sodium.**

82) **Protein foods make you feel full longer and a can help you avoid overeating.**

83) **Free-range animals get more exercise and eat a natural diet, so their meat is usually lower in fat and calories than farm-raised cattle.**

84) Muscle is active tissue, fat is not. The more muscle you have, the more calories you burn. Muscle uses a significant number of calories every day for repair and rebuilding, giving your metabolism a boost even when you're resting. So make sure strengthening exercises (like weight lifting) are part of your workout.

85) Because strengthening exercises work a muscle until it's fatigued, take a day off between strength workouts so your muscles can recover, repair and rebuild.

86) You can workout anywhere you have extra space, in a bedroom, basement, garage, or attic. A set of variable (adjustable) weight dumbbells and a small weight bench don't take up much room and are all you need for a home-based gym.

87) Working out at home has some significant advantages. Your workout takes less time because you don't have to drive back and forth to a fitness facility; and you have the flexibility of dividing your workout into small time segments to fit your day, and working out at home is less expensive.

88) Bear in mind, knowledge and the discipline to workout regularly are far more important than fancy equipment.

89) Avoid injury by warming up and cooling down slowly.

90) Avoid injury by building up exercise intensity gradually over many weeks, months.

91) Stay Busy. Most people will do anything to avoid work, housework, yard work, exercise, etc.   But any kind of work burns a lot more calories than just sitting. Whatever it is you are avoiding – just go and do it!

92)   Buy a pedometer and start walking.   For the average person 2,100 steps amounts to walking about one mile. A Harvard study has shown that 8,000 to 10,000 step per day promotes weight loss.

93) You burn about 100 calories per mile when you walk. Jogging burns about the same 100 calories per mile – but in a shorter time.   And the more you weigh, the more calories you burn during exercise!

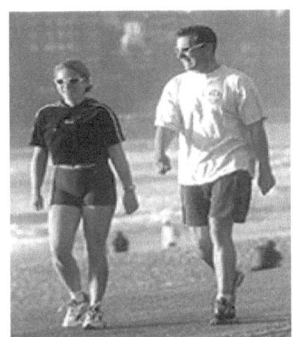

94) Brisk walking not only helps you lose weight but also has many health benefits. So when you walk – don't saunter - walk briskly.

95) For extra exercise, park within walking distance of your destination and walk, and if you're healthy walk up stairs rather than taking an elevator or escalator.

96) For more exercise, take a brisk 15 minute walk around the mall before you start shopping.

97)   For life-long weight control take a vigorous 60 minute walk everyday! That's right – everyday. Make exercise a nonflexible top priority part of your life.

98)   To get and stay fit and help control your weight,

walk everyday and work out with dumbbells for twenty minutes two or three times a week. That's all most people need.

99) Exercise key words are: consistent, persistent, dogged, unyielding, ... Get the point?

100) A common weight-loss fallacy is that you can lose abdominal fat by working your abdominal muscles. This is based on the incorrect belief that fat is eliminated from a particular part of your body if you engage the muscles underneath that layer of fat. No such luck.

101) It's a lot easier to eat 1,000 Calories than it is to burn 1,000 Calories by exercising. So a stroll after dinner won't offset the calories you ingest eating a big meal.

102) It's much easier to stay with an exercise program when it's done in tandem, that is when you exercise with a buddy.

103) Take a daily multi-vitamin/mineral supplement. This is important when you're on a diet – as a kind of insurance policy.

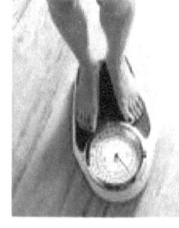 104) Weigh in once a week. There may be times when you might not see a weight loss, often because lost fat is temporarily replaced by water. This condition will gradually be corrected as you continue dieting.

105) To combat a craving think: I'm going to forgo that high-calorie dessert because I want to be around to see my children (or grandchildren) graduate from college.

106) Inevitably, you're going to be faced with a stressful situation. Instead of turning to food for comfort, be prepared with some non-food tactics that work for you, such as listening to music, reading, writing in a journal, or meditating.

107) On a reducing diet, when you lose – you win! You win a much better chance for a longer healthier life, you win a sense of well-being, you win a more attractive appearance – and finally you win a feeling of accomplishment.

108) To prevent or delay the onset of type II diabetes, experts urge the overweight to lose weight and work out regularly. Weight loss helps your body use insulin more efficiently, and exercise helps metabolize excess circulating blood glucose.

109) Take weight Loss one step, one meal, one workout, one day at a time. Just think of where you'll be in a few weeks.

110) Acquire a good low-calorie cookbook. Be sure the recipes cover breakfast, lunch and dinner, and all the recipes contain nutritional information, especially the calories per serving.

111) Obtain a comprehensive food calorie guide such as the excellent U.S.D.A. Home and Garden Bulletin No. 72: "Nutritive Value of Foods," which can be downloaded online at no cost.

112) And get a scientifically sound and effective weight control book to help you lose weight in a safe and healthy manner. Consider NoPaperPress, with its extensive line of weight control, nutrition and exercise eBooks written by experts for sensible adults. No fad diets here!

113) Plan to be on a diet the rest of your life. Not necessarily a weight-reducing diet. Hopefully, at some point you'll just be maintaining your weight. But you will still need to continue to make good healthy food choices – and not slip back to your old eating habits.

Weight Maintenance Tips

Researchers have found that most people can lose weight on almost any diet. The key concern is whether the weight loss can be maintained. In fact, the real challenge is not getting people to lose weight but helping them keep it off. Few, if any, weight control programs have been successful at helping people maintain their weight over the long term.

The following tips are offered to help you maintain your weight. Use the tips that apply to you and can best make it easier for you to succeed. Good luck!

114) The two key issues in weight maintenance are: Preventing the regaining of lost weight after a diet, and preventing weight gain as you age.

115) If you are overweight start on a weight loss diet now because it will only become more difficult to lose weight as you get older.

116) If your caloric intake is constant over the years you will slowly gain weight as you age. This is because your metabolic rate decreases as you age, and most older people also tend to not be as active.

117) Understand that the only sure way to slim down for keeps is to eat less and exercise more. There are no safe short cuts or miracle methods for maintaining your weight.

118) Successful weight loss and subsequent weight maintenance requires knowledge, desire and discipline. Avoid the latest fad diets. Instead, take the time to develop a true understanding of weight control and then change your eating and activity habits accordingly.

119) Consistently choose healthy foods, avoid harmful foods and large portions and exercise regularly. Nothing else will work in the long haul.

120) Experts agree that whether you are trying to lose weight or just maintain your weight, it's calories that count. It doesn't matter what foods the calories are from – to lose weight you must eat fewer calories than you burn. Calories count!   Not carbs, not Weight Watchers points. Calories – period!

121) Weight control can be thought of as supply and demand. You lose weight if you supply your body with fewer calories than your activities demand. (In this case, your body uses energy you stored as fat to make up the calorie difference.)

122) Weight loss occurs when your food energy intake is less than the total energy you expend. This difference in calories is referred to as your calorie deficit.

122) After any diet, your lower body weight requires fewer calories to function. In other words, your lower body weight results in a slower metabolism.

123) Within five years, most dieters regain every pound they have lost. Why? In most cases it's because after losing weight most people eventually revert to their pre-diet eating and exercising habits, and this inevitably leads to their regaining the weight they lost – and often more.

124) The fact is the less you weigh, the less you need to eat to maintain your lower weight. Without some lifestyle modifications, if you are like the average adult you will regain every pound you have lost. It's a fact that 95 percent of dieters regain all the weight they lost back and often more!

125)   A study, published in the Annals of Internal Medicine, followed 4,000 people for three decades suggests that in the long term, 90 percent of men and 70 percent of women will become overweight (BMI greater than or equal to 25). In fact, half of the men and women in the study, had made it well into adulthood without a weight problem, but ultimately also became overweight and a third became obese.

126) Why does this happen? When people reach their mid to late twenties, they slowly start to lose muscle and add fat as part of the natural aging process.

127) So as you age your muscle mass slowly deteriorates and is replaced by fat. But muscle is active tissue and requires lots of energy (calories) for growth and repair; whereas, fat is basically inactive and uses very few calories to subsist.

128)   In fact, your metabolism decreases about 10 percent every decade. For the average adult, the result of a slowing metabolism is a weight gain of

almost 2 pounds every year. To offset this, you need to cut back on the calories you consume, or increase your exercise, or both, or the excess calories will add up and so will your weight!

129) A study published in the American Journal of Preventive Medicine, surveyed adults from 1999 to 2002 who were overweight or obese and lost at least 10 percent of their maximum weight. The study authors found some common factors associated with those who regained their weight.

130) Those who regained lost weight spent four hours or more per day in front of a TV or computer. Too much TV or computer time usually means these people are probably getting very little exercise.

131) Those who regained lost a lot of weight (at least 20 percent of their maximum weight) in a short time. Because it takes time to establish a new lifestyle that supports weight maintenance, people who lost weight quickly, may not have had the time to acquire the skills needed to maintain their lower weight.

132) Those who regained started to regain weight soon after they stopped dieting. Losing weight too fast, either by fad or extreme dieting, can leave people feeling deprived and often ends up triggering binges that go on until the lost weight is regained.

133) The National Weight Control Registry studied people who had lost at least 30 pounds and kept it off for more than a year. They found that although people lost weight differently, they kept it off similarly. The following are some characteristics of the successful maintainers.

134) Most successful maintainers eat a moderately low-fat diet.

135) Successful maintainers monitor portion sizes.

136) Most maintainers eat breakfast every day.

137) Most are physically active, with walking their most common exercise and they walk for about an hour every day. (And these people probably aren't watching hours of TV daily.)

138) Most successful maintainers find pleasure in their healthier lifestyle and diet-free living.

139) One dilemma for dieters is judging portion size. It makes no sense to worry about whether a cut of lean meat has 70 or 80 Calories per ounce if you have no idea whether the portion you are eating weighs four or ten ounces. To be successful, learn to estimate portion sizes with reasonable accuracy.

140) Judging the weight of meat or poultry is one of the most important parts of any diet. As a guide, four ounces of meat or poultry is about the size of a slice of bread: 4 x 4 x ¼ inch.

141) Eat the low-cal items on your plate first. Start with a broth soup, then the salad and veggies. By the time you get to the higher calorie meat and starch you'll be almost full and will eat less of them.

142) Steaming in a microwave is an excellent way to cook veggies so they retain nutrients. Another advantage is that steaming adds no fat (calories) or sodium.

143) Protein foods make you feel full longer and a can help you avoid overeating.

144) Plan to be on a diet the rest of your life. Not necessarily a weight-reducing diet. But you will still need to continue to make good healthy food choices – and not slip back to your old eating habits.

145) Finally, get a scientifically sound and effective weight control book to help you maintain your weight in a safe and healthy manner. Consider WEIGHT MAINTENANCE - U.S. Edition by Vincent Antonetti, PhD, also published by NoPaperPress, and absolutely the best weight maintenance book on the market.

Healthy Eating Tips

Use the tips that apply to you and can best lead you to a healthier way of eating. Good luck!

146) The diet of most Americans is not very healthy. We consume too many calories and too much saturated fat, trans fat, cholesterol, added sugars and salt.

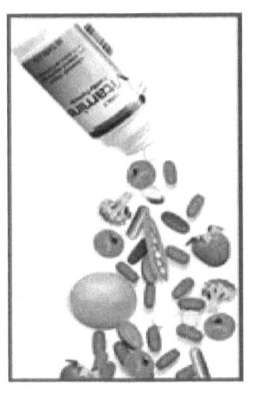

147) Proteins, carbohydrates and fats are nutrients. Vitamins and minerals are called micronutrients because they are present in foods in much smaller amounts than nutrients. Both are essential to human life.

148) Despite the fact that most adults can get all the vitamins and

minerals they need by merely consuming a variety of nutritious foods, many physicians recommend a daily multi-vitamin/mineral supplement as a kind of insurance policy.

149) Many adults over 50 are unable to absorb vitamin B12 in food. People over 50 are able to absorb the synthetic vitamin B12 added to fortified foods and dietary supplements.

150) Phytonutrients, the compounds that give fruits and vegetables their color, are also found in whole grains, dried beans, nuts and seeds. They have many beneficial qualities such as reducing inflammation, acting against viruses, and helping reduce the risk some chronic ailments.

151) Nutritionists define a "junk food" as one that offers little if any essential nutrients – except calories and when eaten it replaces more important foods.

152) In the U.S., we consume more than 100 pounds of sugar per year per person, totaling an unhealthy, nutritionally empty, 500 Calories per day. This large intake of sugar leads to obvious ills, such as obesity and tooth decay.

153) Sugar should be used sparingly by people with low calorie needs and in moderation by most other healthy adults.

154) Contrary to what many believe, the latest scientific evidence indicate diets high in sugar do not cause diabetes. Rather, the evidence indicates that adult-onset diabetes occurs most often in those who are overweight.

155) Thinking about using honey rather than sugar? Honey has about 21 calories per teaspoon while sugar has 15. And the vitamin and mineral content of honey is very low.

156) Free-range animals get more exercise and eat a natural diet, so their meat is usually lower in fat and calories than farm-raised cattle.

157) There is no conclusive evidence that shows that organic food is more nutritious than conventionally grown non-organic food.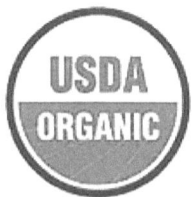

158) But in the view of many nutritionists, if you can afford it, buy local and organic. You don't have to buy organic across the board because not all organic-labeled products offer added health value.

159) It's worth buying organic for the "dirty dozen": peaches, strawberries, nectarines, apples, spinach, celery, pears, sweet bell peppers, cherries, potatoes, lettuce, and imported grapes. These fragile fruits and vegetables often require more pesticides to fight off bugs

160) Studies have shown vegetarian diets significantly lower the risk of colon cancer, heart disease, high blood pressure and other diseases.

161) Many health care professionals think that eating a healthy vegetarian diet is one of the best things you can do for your short-term and long-term health. But a vegetarian diet must be carefully planned.

162) Drink lots of water – about 8 glasses per day. Try adding a slice of lemon to make it more interesting.

163) Know your daily caloric allowance whether you are trying to maintain your weight or are on a reducing diet. (Again see "Total Fitness - U.S. Edition" by NoPaperPress where you can determine your daily caloric allowance using unique Weight Maintenance tables.)

164) Eat a variety of foods within your caloric allowance, and use the USDA Pyramid to shape your eating patterns. Remember variety is the basis of a nutritious diet.

165) When possible, select fresh and natural foods and whole-grain products. Avoid chemical preservatives and additives, artificial and imitation foods, refined and processed foods, and foods that are comprised of "nutritionally-empty calories."

166) Fiber is an important part of a healthy diet. According to the Harvard University School of Public Health, adequate fiber intake reduces your risk of developing various conditions, including heart disease, diabetes, diverticular disease, and constipation.

167) When you eat fiber, it simply passes straight through, untouched by but aiding your digestive system. Zero calories absorbed!

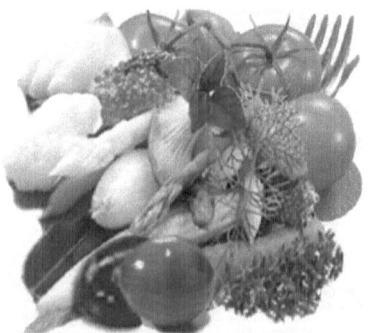

168) Adults should get a least 20 to 35 grams of dietary fiber per day. The best sources are fresh fruits and vegetables, nuts and legumes, and whole-grain foods.

169) For a delicious fiber boost in your diet, try roasted veggies like zucchini and red peppers over whole-grain pasta.

170) Most berries (such as blueberries, raspberries) have even more fiber than a comparable weight of most any other fruit.

171) In the United States, for a food to be labeled "whole grain" it must contain more than 51 percent whole grain by weight.

172) Most Americans consume too much sodium (salt). The U.S. Department of Agriculture Dietary Guidelines recommend that healthy adults limit sodium intake to 2,400 mg per day. (One teaspoon of salt contains about 2,300 mg of sodium.)

173) Before you buy, read and understand the labels on food packages.

174) Protein foods make you feel full longer and a can help you avoid overeating.

175) Nearly every animal food, including dairy products, eggs, meat, poultry and fish are complete proteins because they contain all eight-essential amino acids. Soy is the only plant-based food that has all eight essential-amino acids.

176) Plant-based protein sources lack one or more essential amino acids. Legumes, grains, nuts, and seeds are incomplete proteins.

177) For a complete-protein meal, simply eat any of the incomplete proteins with another but different incomplete protein. Complete proteins result when

legumes are eaten with grains, or legumes with nuts or seeds, or grains with nuts or seeds.

178) Harvard Medical School studied egg consumption among 120,000 health professionals with normal cholesterol levels and reported no link between eating eggs and heart disease or stroke.

179) All fish are relatively low-calorie foods and are good sources of protein and fat-soluble vitamins A and D.

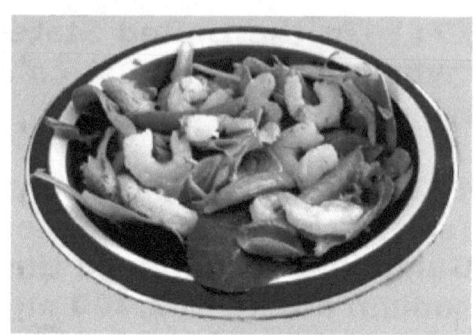

180) Oily cold-water fish such as wild salmon, sardines, herring, mackerel and tuna are high in omega-3 essential-fatty acid. Trout also has comparatively high omega-3 content.

181) A downside to eating fish is that some fish are contaminated with mercury, PCBs, dioxins and other environmental pollutants.

182) Large predatory fish such as shark, swordfish, king mackerel and tilefish have the highest concentration of mercury and other environmental contaminates. U.S. Food and Drug Administration advises adults to eat no more than six ounces of high-mercury fish per week.

183) Skinless white-meat chicken and turkey are relatively low calorie, low fat, low cholesterol foods that are powerful sources of high-quality protein, vitamin B_6, riboflavin, niacin, phosphorus and potassium.

184) All soy foods contain a significant amount of plant-based complete protein and omega-3 fatty acid as well as vitamin E, potassium, iron and folate.

185) Carbohydrates provide your body with its basic fuel, the energy your cells need to survive, as well as essential vitamins and minerals, fiber, and other beneficial compounds that promote good health.

186) Fruit and milk are loaded with natural sugar (a carb). But the natural sugar comes with vitamins, minerals (as well as fiber when you eat fruit); whereas the simple sugars in candy, for instance, are nothing but nutritionally-empty calories.

187) Simple sugars require little digestion. When you eat a sweet food, such as a candy bar, your blood sugar level rises rapidly. In response, your pancreas secretes a large amount of insulin. The large insulin response tends to cause your blood sugar to fall to levels that are too low, and in about three hours you feel lethargic and hungry.

188) A relatively new system, called the glycemic index (GI), measures the effect a carbohydrate has on your blood sugar – quantifying how rapidly and to what level your blood sugar rises after you eat a food containing carbohydrates.

189) A candy bar, which is digested rapidly has a high GI and causes an almost immediate jump in your blood sugar; whereas, lentil soup is digested more slowly and has a low GI.

190) The blood lipids cholesterol and triglyceride are found in the plaque on the walls of clogged arteries.

191) **Desirable readings for healthy individuals are:** Total cholesterol level should be less than 200 mg/dl; High-density cholesterol (HDL) should be greater than 40 mg/dl; Low-density cholesterol (LDL) should be less than 130 mg/dl; Triglyceride reading should be less than 150 mg/dl.

192) The latest research seems to show that the total amount of fat in the diet may not be strongly linked with disease. What appears to matter is the type of fat in your diet.

193) Limit your intake of saturated fats. Eat meat less often and fish and poultry more often, and use fat-free or low-fat milk and milk products.

194) Do not eat foods containing partially-hydrogenated vegetable oil because they are high in trans fats. This includes commercially prepared baked goods, snack foods, and processed foods, including most fast foods.

195) Monounsaturated fats "good fats" are derived from plant sources, such as vegetable oils, nuts, and seeds. This type of fat is found in high concentrations in canola, olive and peanut oils.

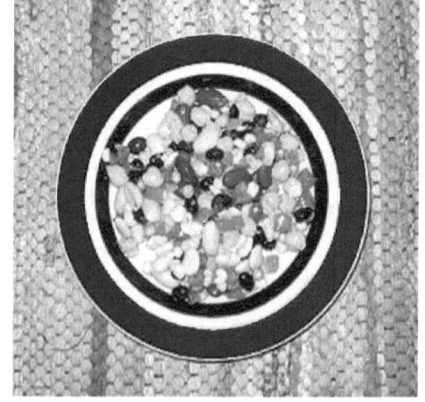

196) Polyunsaturated fats are also "good fats" and are derived from plant sources, such as vegetable oils, nuts, and seeds, and are in high concentrations in sunflower, soybean and corn oils.

197) Essential-Fatty Acids are class of polyunsaturated fatty acids that our body cannot create. These fats must be obtained from the food you eat and fall into two groups: omega-3 and omega-6.

198) Omega-3 fatty acids, thought to be heart-protective, are relatively hard to find. Foods high in omega-3 fatty acids are walnuts, tofu, flax seeds and oily fish (salmon, mackerel, sardines, trout and albacore tuna).

199) Omega-6 fatty acids, on the other hand, are more common, easier to find, and are in most oils including sunflower, soybean and corn oils.

200) According to a study published in the Journal of Food Chemistry, broccoli, spinach, kale, Brussels sprouts and other dark green vegetables have the highest cancer-fighting potential found in produce. And all are super-low calorie foods.

201) It's a lot easier to eat 1,000 Calories than it is to burn 1,000 Calories by exercising. So a stroll after dinner won't offset the calories you ingest eating a big meal.

202) Consistently choose healthy foods, avoid harmful foods and large portions and exercise regularly. Nothing else will control your weight over the long haul.

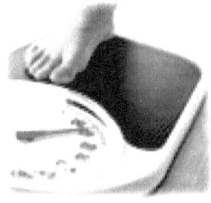

203) Your body weight fluctuates two to three pounds daily. Your weight is lowest before breakfast and highest in the evening before retiring.

204) Finally, get a scientifically sound and effective nutrition book to help you eat a safe and healthy manner. Consider NoPaperPress, with its extensive line of nutrition, weight control and exercise eBooks written by experts for sensible adults.

Life-Long Fitness Tips

The following are offered to help you get physically fit in a healthy and effective manner. Use the tips that apply to you and that can best help you succeed. Good luck!

205) To get fit and stay fit, exercise regularly, do not smoke, practice good nutrition, maintain a proper weight level, and have periodic medical checkups.

206) Benefits of being fit: Lower blood pressure; a stronger and more efficient heart; supple and young arteries; a higher metabolic rate; larger more powerful muscles with more definition, and stronger bones.

207) When you're physically fit, you'll look and feel younger than your chronological age and you'll probably live longer too.

208) You should have a medical exam, before starting a physical fitness program. This is especially important if you are overweight, if you have been inactive, if you have a history of medical problems, or if you are 40 or older.

209) Remember to discuss your physical fitness plan and your short-term and long-term goals with your doctor.

210) Before you start a physical fitness program you should know your current fitness level. Assessing your current level in areas such as aerobic (cardio) capacity, strength, flexibility, body-fat, will help you determine what you should emphasize and help you set realistic goals.

211) A good measure of your cardio-respiratory fitness, is the volume of oxygen per minute per kilogram of body weight (called VO2max) you can process during hard exercise.

212) A good self-assessment test for VO2max is the Rockport Walking Test. After walking a mile as rapidly as you can, you record your pulse and the time to complete the walk. You then convert your time and pulse into VO2max using formulae and a table in "Total Fitness – U.S. Edition" (by NoPaperPress.com).

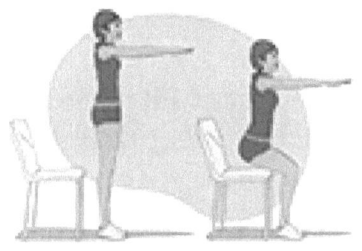

213) Self-assessment strength tests include a Push-up Test, a Sit-up Test, and a Squat Test. For descriptions of the tests and to interpret your test results and see how fit you are, see "Total Fitness – U.S. Edition".

214) The standard self-assessment test for flexibility is the "Sit and Reach Test." Again see "Total Fitness – U.S. Edition."

215) Exercise physiologists consider the percentage of body fat compared to total body weight a critical measure of fitness, and contend, from the standpoint

of good health, that men should have no more than 20 percent body fat and women no more than 23 percent body fat.

216) Muscle is active tissue, fat is not. The more muscle you have, the more calories you burn. Muscle uses a significant number of calories every day for repair and rebuilding giving your metabolism a boost even when you're resting. So make sure strengthening exercises (like weight lifting) are part of your workout.

217) Stay Busy. Most people will do anything to avoid work, housework, yard work, exercise, etc. But any kind of work burns a lot more calories than just sitting. Whatever it is you are avoiding – just go and do it!

218) Consider anytime you have to lift, bend, reach, walk as an opportunity to burn additional calories and as an extension of your formal workout.

219) Get a good chart (like the one in Total Fitness - U.S. Edition) that lists how many calories are burned for different activities – depending on what you weigh.

220) Engage in leisure activities such as dancing, bowling and gardening more often. They can be enjoyable and provide added exercise.

221) If you work at a desk, stand up and stretch two or three times a day, read standing up, etcetera.

222) If you've been inactive for some time, rather than starting with one of the more strenuous exercises, you should initially confine yourself to walking until you can easily walk two miles at a brisk pace. When you reach this stage more strenuous exercises can be attempted if desired.

223) Some sports medicine physicians contend that if you are badly overweight you should limit your exercise to walking until you are less than 25 percent overweight.

224) An exercise buddy can make exercise more enjoyable and can help you get going and keep going on days when you might otherwise quit.

225) On the other hand, an exercise partner probably means that you now have the schedules of two busy people to contend with and plan around, which can at times actually hinder your workout.

226) You must be open to rearranging your priorities to fit exercise into your daily life.

227) To improve muscle tone and overall fitness, feel good and stay healthy, you should exercise at least five days per week, day after day, week after week, year after year – for as long as you are physically able.

228) Remember exercise key words: consistent, determined, steady, persistent, dogged, unswerving, gritty, single-minded. Consistent!

229) Walking is a wonderful exercise. It's an exercise you can do anywhere, that you can do well into your old age, that you can do outdoors or indoors, and that requires no special equipment

other than a good comfortable pair of walking shoes. Whereas, joining and working out at a fitness center can be relatively expensive.

230)   Buy a pedometer and start walking.   For the average person 2,100 steps amounts to walking about one mile. A Harvard study has shown that 8,000 to 10,000 step per day promotes weight loss.

231) Walk to burn calories and lose weight. You burn about 100 calories for each mile that you walk. Jogging burns about the same 100 calories per mile – but in a shorter time.

232) 160 lb person (man or woman) walking at 3.5 mph burns about 320 Calories in one hour.

234) Look for opportunities to walk, such as walking to a local store rather than driving, walking the course if you play golf, and mowing your lawn.

235) For extra exercise, park within walking distance of your destination and walk, and if you're healthy walk up stairs rather than taking an elevator or escalator.

236) For more exercise, take a brisk 15 minute walk around the mall before you start shopping.

237)   For life-long weight control take a vigorous 30 to 60 minute walk everyday! That's right – everyday. Make exercise a nonflexible top priority part of your life.

238) Aerobic (cardio) exercises, such as jogging, swimming, cycling, brisk walking, skipping rope, and many others, are typically deep breathing and

continuous, with rhythmic and repetitive contractions of your large muscle groups.

239) Most aerobic exercises have one thing in common: they make you work hard and require you to process a great deal of oxygen.

240) If you want to strengthen your heart and lungs, improve your aerobic capacity and burn a lot of calories select a vigorous aerobic activity such as jogging.

241) A classic aerobic exercise routine consists of a warm up, your main exercise, and a cool down period.

242) If you jog, always choose endurance over intensity; i.e., choose distance rather than speed, choose to jog longer rather than faster.

243) If you decide to exercise outdoors you should also have an alternate indoor activity, an activity you can fall back on in bad weather.

244) If you jog outside early in the morning before work, you may want to purchase a treadmill for use at home on days when it is either too hot, too cold or the weather is just bad.

245) Be aware that the pounding your body gets

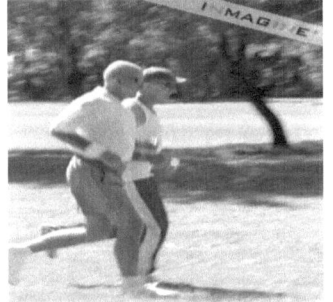

from jogging usually takes its toll over time. Many joggers have recurring, nagging injuries, particularly to their legs and feet.

246) If you start to suffer chronic injuries, try other high-intensity aerobic exercises for

which your body might be better suited such as cycling, a rowing machine, etc.

247) You if you cannot converse comfortably with a partner while you are walking briskly, jogging, cycling, etc. A feeling of having worked hard is fine, sweating is good, but not a feeling of undo fatigue.

248) Potentially serious problems are signaled if you experience any of the following during or after exercise: Symptoms include but are not limited to difficulty breathing; abnormal heart action such as irregular heart rhythm; pain or pressure in the middle of your chest; pain in an arm or your neck; dizziness, fainting or lightheadedness; severe exhaustion; sudden loss of coordination; or confusion. If you experience any of these symptoms, stop exercising immediately and get medical help.

249) Another definition of the beneficial yet safe aerobic exercise region is referred to as the "Target Training Zone," which is determined by monitoring your pulse. The idea is to raise your pulse through exercise to a specific range (the target training zone) and hold it there for an extended period to obtain a cardiovascular benefit.

250) The American College of Sports Medicine recommends an exercise heart rate of 60 to 90 percent of your maximum heart rate should be maintained for about 30 to 45 minutes three to five days per week to become reasonably fit.

251) To monitor the intensity of your exercise, you should occasionally stop during your workout and take your pulse immediately. (To find your pulse,

quickly place the tips of two fingers on a carotid artery in your neck. Then count the beats for ten seconds and multiply by six.)

252) The ideal exercise temperature range is about 40 to 85°F with a wind speed less than 15 mph.

253) When you engage in vigorous exercise, your body generates a great deal of heat. On hot humid summer days, your body temperature can rise from 98.6°F up to 101°F. (A body temperature of 105°F is life threatening.)

254) In hot weather, be guided by the Heat Index, or apparent temperature, which combines the effects of air (dry bulb) temperature and relative humidity.

255) Before exercising outdoors in hot weather, check your local weather forecast. If the forecast does not incorporate the heat index, you can use the forecasted air temperature and relative humidity to determine a heat index value using tables, such as those in "Total Fitness - U.S. Edition" by Vincent Antonetti, PhD - published by NoPaperPress.

256) Exercising when the Heat Index is 90 to 105°F can result in muscle cramps and/or heat exhaustion. The much more dangerous heat stroke is possible when the Heat Index is over 105°F.

257) Unless you are relatively young and in very good physical condition, it's not a good idea to engage in vigorous outdoor exercise when the heat index is over 90°F.

258) Drinking water is important for good health, but it's even more important on hot days while you

are exercising. During vigorous exercise, you can lose one to two quarts of water
per hour in sweat, so when you exercise it's essential to use common sense and stay hydrated.

259) Many people exercise outdoors at temperatures well below 40°F. To an exerciser, cold weather is usually less dangerous than extremely hot weather to an exerciser – but definitely is not risk-free.

260) Very low ambient temperatures combined with the wind increase the amount of heat leaving your body. As the wind speed increases, the temperature of any exposed skin drops
even further.

261) In cold weather, be guided by the Wind Chill Temperature Index which is a measure of the relative discomfort due to combined cold temperature and wind.

262) Potentially serious consequences of very low wind-chill temperatures are frostbite, hypothermia and heart attack.

63) At wind-chill temperature of approximately 10°F exercising outdoors becomes increasingly uncomfortable. Even if you are an outdoor enthusiast, at this wind chill you may want to think about changing to an indoor exercise.

264) At a wind-chill temperature of approximately -17°F the risk of frostbite starts to increase.

265) Before exercising outdoors in cold weather, check your local weather forecast. It's not a good idea to exercise outdoors when the wind-chill temperature is below -20°F

because any exposed skin will freeze in about 10 minutes.

266) If you insist on working out in very hot or cold weather, always let someone know when and where you will be exercising and when you are planning to return.

267) Your body has approximately 650 muscles that account for more than half your body weight.

268) As you age you loose muscle mass, your bone density decreases and you lose strength. Exercises like weight lifting strengthen your muscles, bones and joints and also reduce your risk of developing osteoporosis.

269) If you want to become physically stronger choose one of the strength-building exercises such as weight lifting.

270) Because strengthening exercises work a muscle until it's fatigued, take a day off between strength workouts for your muscles to recover, repair and rebuild.

271) in a bedroom, basement, garage, or attic. A set of variable (adjustable) weight dumbbells and a small weight bench don't take up much room and are all you need for a home-based gym.

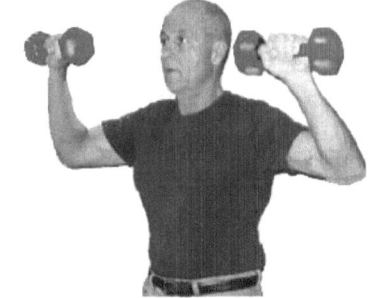

272) Working out at home has some significant advantages. Your workout takes less time because you don't have to drive back and

forth to a fitness facility; and you have the flexibility of dividing your workout into small time segments to fit your day, and working out at home is less expensive.

273) Bear in mind, knowledge and the discipline to workout regularly are far more important than fancy equipment.

274) When you start weight training, rather than purchase an entire set of weights, buy just enough dumbbell weight so that you can do a military press five times.

275) Never hold your breath during weight training. This can cause your blood pressure to get dangerously high. Rather, breathe naturally and try to exhale during a lift.

276) If you only miss working out for a day or two, you can just pick up where you left off as if nothing happened. If you miss a week or more, you probably have lost some of your fitness gains and might have to resume at a somewhat lower exercising-intensity level. Listen to your body.

277) A common weight-loss fallacy is that you can lose abdominal fat by working your abdominal muscles. This is based on the incorrect belief that fat is eliminated from a particular part of your body if you engage the muscles underneath that layer of fat. No such luck.

279) Avoid injury by building up exercise intensity gradually over many weeks, months.

280) Avoid injury by waiting two hours after a meal before you start exercising.

281) Avoid injury by waiting 30 minutes after exercising before you eat.

282) Avoid injury by using safety and protective equipment as appropriate, such as helmet when you bicycle, and goggles when you play handball, squash or racquetball.

283) Avoid injury by warming up and cooling down slowly.

284) Avoid injury by not increasing the difficulty of any activity (e.g., your walking or jogging distance, the amount of weight you lift) by more than 10 percent per week.

285) Avoid injury by jogging on softer surfaces such as a level grass field, a dirt path, or a running track.

286) Many minor leg injuries of the muscles and joints can be treated using the well-known R.I.C.E. method, i.e., rest, ice, compression, elevation.

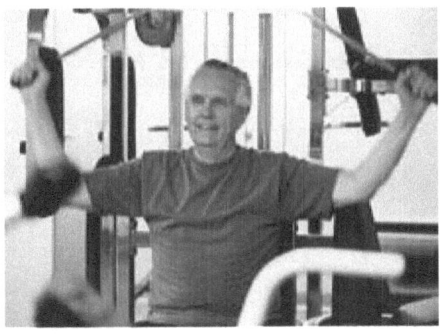

287) If you are, attend an orientation session before you use any unfamiliar exercise equipment. Otherwise, read the operating instructions carefully and ask someone qualified to help you.

288) The majority of exercise physiologists feel that sports drinks are unnecessary for most people, and that plain water, along with the salt in the food we

eat, are all that is needed to replenish the water and sodium lost during <u>moderate</u> exercise.

289) It's a lot easier to eat 1,000 Calories than it is to burn 1,000 Calories by exercising. So a stroll after dinner won't offset the calories you ingest eating a big meal.

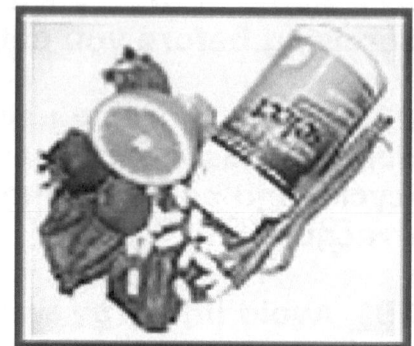

290) Keep a daily log to record your progress. For some people it really works wonders.

291)   To get and stay fit and help control your weight, walk everyday and work out with dumbbells for twenty minutes two or three times a week. That's all most people need.

10 Best Tips

The most important tips from each of the four categories are listed here.

292) Given a male and female, the same age, weight, activity level and on the same reducing diet, the man will lose weight faster than the woman. This is because most women have less muscle and therefore lower basal metabolic rates than most men. Hence, in general, a woman must eat less than a man to lose the same amount of weight.

293) Given two individuals, the same gender, weight and activity level, the younger person will lose weight faster than the older person. So if you are overweight start on a weight loss diet now because it will only become more difficult to lose weight as you get older.

294) "Eat Slowly." This is especially vital when you're trying to lose weight. If you're someone who eats fast, you're not giving yourself a chance to feel full. While everyone else is still eating, you either sit and pick, or you have seconds, taking in extra calories you could avoid if you would just slow down.

295) Experts agree that whether you are trying to lose weight or just maintain your weight, it's calories that count.   It doesn't matter what foods the calories are from – to lose weight you must eat fewer calories than you burn. Calories count!   Not carbs, not Weight Watchers points. Calories – period!

296) The two key issues in weight maintenance are: Preventing the regaining of lost weight after a diet, and preventing weight gain as you age.

297) Most successful weight maintainers are physically active, with walking their most common exercise and they walk for about an hour every day. (And these people probably aren't watching hours of TV daily.)

298) Most successful maintainers find pleasure in their healthier lifestyle and diet-free living.

299) Eat a variety of foods within your caloric allowance, and use the USDA Pyramid to shape your eating patterns. Remember variety is the basis of a nutritious diet.

300) To get fit and stay fit, exercise regularly, do not smoke, practice good nutrition, maintain a proper weight level, and have periodic medical checkups.

301) Before you start a physical fitness program you should know your current fitness level. Assessing your current level in areas such as aerobic (cardio) capacity, strength, flexibility, body-fat, will help you determine what you should emphasize and help you set realistic goals.

Disclaimer: This work offers general fitness, exercise, nutrition and weight control information. It is not a medical manual and the authors do not claim to be medically qualified. The material in this book is not intended to be a substitute for medical counseling. Everyone should have a medical checkup before beginning a physical fitness program. Moreover, the physician conducting the medical exam should be made aware of and should approve the specific physical fitness program planned. Additionally, while the authors and publisher have made every effort to ensure the accuracy of the information in this book, they make no representations or warranties regarding its accuracy or completeness. Further, neither the authors nor publisher assume liability for any medical problems that might result from applying the methods in this book, or for any loss of profit, or any other commercial damages, including but not limited to special, incidental, consequential or other damages, and any such liability is hereby expressly disclaimed.